The Quick Mediterranean Delicacies

Fast, Delicious and On a Budget Recipes to Boost Your Brain

Alison Russell

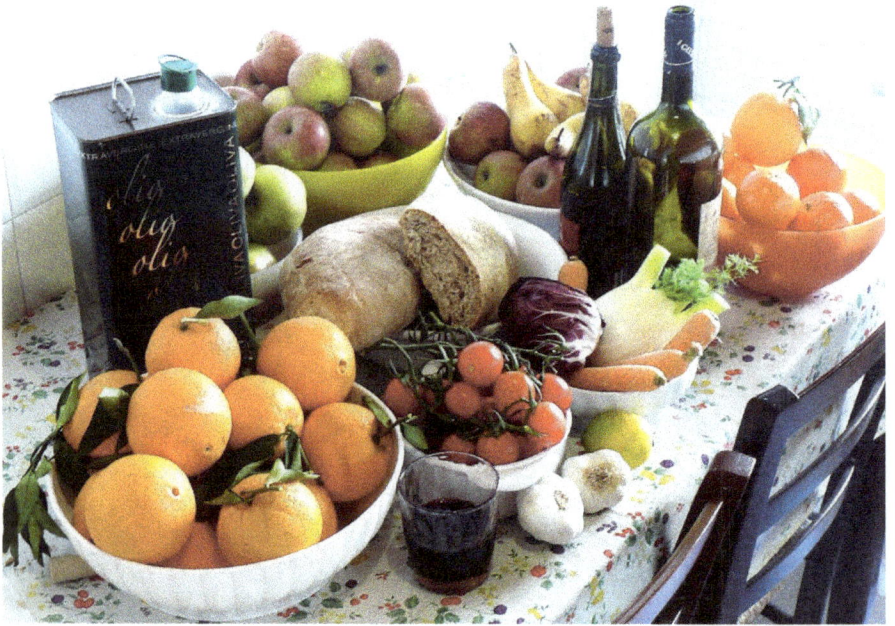

Table of contents

Beans, Grains, and Pastas

Cumin Quinoa Pilaf

Prep time: 5 minutes | Cook time: 5 minutes | Serves 2

2 tablespoons extra virgin olive oil

2 teaspoons ground cumin

2 cloves garlic, minced

2 teaspoons turmeric

3 cups water

Salt, to taste

2 cups quinoa, rinsed

1 handful parsley, chopped

1. Press the Sauté button to heat your Instant Pot.
2. Once hot, add the oil and garlic to the pot, stir and cook for 1 minute.
3. Add water, quinoa, cumin, turmeric, and salt, stirring well.
4. Lock the lid. Select the Manual mode and set the cooking time for 1 minute at High Pressure.
5. When the timer beeps, perform a natural pressure release for 10 minutes, then release any remaining pressure. Carefully remove the lid.
6. Fluff the quinoa with a fork. Season with more salt, if needed.

7. Sprinkle the chopped parsley on top and serve.

Per Serving

calories: 384 | fat: 12.3g | protein: 12.8g | carbs: 57.4g | fiber: 6.9g | sodium: 448mg

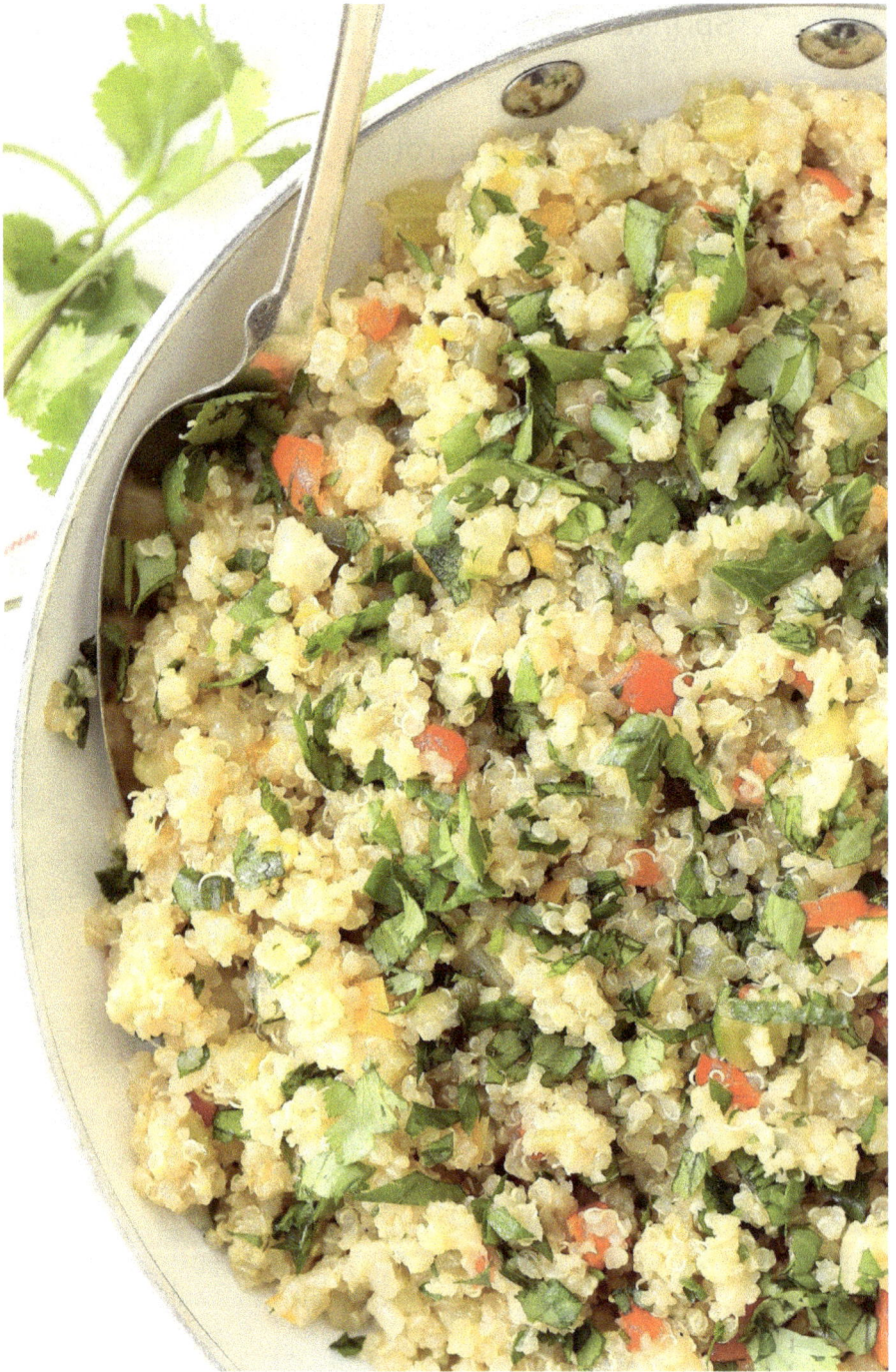

Mint Brown Rice

Prep time: 5 minutes | Cook time: 22 minutes | Serves 2

2 cloves garlic, minced

¼ cup chopped fresh mint, plus more for garnish

1 tablespoon chopped dried chives

1 cup short- or long-grain brown rice

1½ cups water or low-sodium vegetable broth

½ to 1 teaspoon sea salt

1. Place the garlic, mint, chives, rice, and water in the Instant Pot. Stir to combine.
2. Secure the lid. Select the Manual mode and set the cooking time for 22 minutes at High Pressure.
3. Once cooking is complete, do a natural pressure release for 10 minutes, then release any remaining pressure. Carefully open the lid.
4. Add salt to taste and serve garnished with more mint.

Per Serving

calories: 514 | fat: 6.6g | protein: 20.7g | carbs: 80.4g | fiber: 3.3g | sodium: 786mg

Rice and Sweet Potato Pilaf

Prep time: 15 minutes | Cook time: 10 minutes | Serves 4 to 6

2 tablespoons extra-virgin olive oil

1 onion, chopped fine

½ teaspoon table salt

2 garlic cloves, minced

1½ teaspoons ground turmeric

1 teaspoon ground coriander

⅛ teaspoon cayenne pepper

2 cups chicken broth

12 ounces (340 g) sweet potato, peeled, quartered lengthwise, and sliced ½ inch thick

½ preserved lemon, pulp and white pith removed, rind rinsed and minced (2 tablespoons)

½ cup shelled pistachios, toasted and chopped

¼ cup fresh cilantro leaves

¼ cup pomegranate seeds

1½ cups long-grain

white rice, rinsed

1. Using highest Sauté function, heat oil in Instant Pot until shimmering. Add onion and salt and cook until onion is softened, about 5 minutes. Stir in garlic, turmeric, coriander, and cayenne and cook until fragrant, about 30 seconds. Stir in broth, rice, and sweet potato.

2. Lock lid in place and close pressure release valve. Select Manual function and cook for 4 minutes. Turn off Instant Pot and quick release pressure. Carefully remove lid, allowing steam to escape away from you.

3. Add preserved lemon and gently fluff rice with fork to combine. Lay clean dish towel over pot, replace lid, and let sit for 5 minutes. Season with salt and pepper to taste. Transfer to serving dish and sprinkle with pistachios, cilantro, and pomegranate seeds. Serve.

Per Serving

calories: 698 | fat: 22.8g | protein: 36.8g | carbs: 85.5g | fiber: 5.9g | sodium: 802mg

Shrimp and Asparagus Risotto

Prep time: 15 minutes | Cook time: 58 minutes | Serves 4

1 tablespoon olive oil

1 pound (454 g) asparagus, trimmed and roughly chopped

1 cup spinach, chopped

1½ cups mushrooms, chopped

1 cup rice, rinsed and drained

1¼ cups chicken broth

¾ cup milk

1 tablespoon coconut oil

16 shrimp, cleaned and deveined

Salt and ground black pepper, to taste

¾ cup Parmesan cheese, shredded

1. Warm the oil on Sauté. Add spinach, mushrooms and asparagus and Sauté for 10 minutes until cooked through. Press Cancel. Add rice, milk and chicken broth to the pot as you stir.

2. Seal the lid, press Multigrain and cook for 40 minutes on High Pressure. Do a quick release, open the lid and put the rice on a serving plate.

3. Take back the empty pot to the pressure cooker, add coconut oil and press Sauté. Add shrimp and cook each side for 4 minutes until cooked through and turns pink. Set shrimp over rice, add pepper and salt for seasoning. Serve topped with shredded Parmesan cheese.

Per Serving

calories: 385 | fat: 14.3g | protein: 16.5g | carbs: 48.4g | fiber: 4.1g | sodium: 771mg

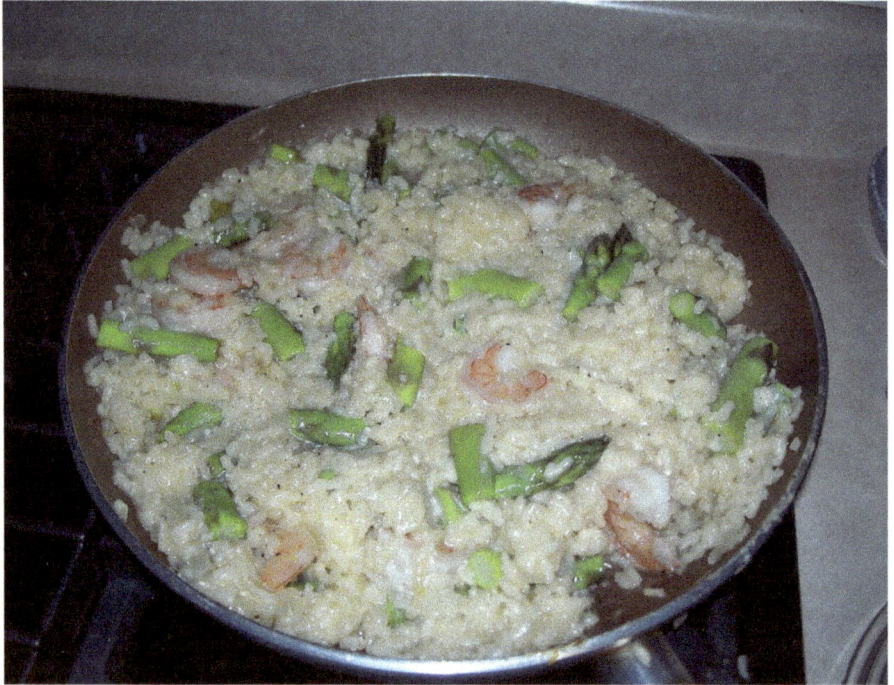

Pancetta with Garbanzo Beans

Prep time: 10 minutes | Cook time: 38 minutes | Serves 6

3 strips pancetta	½ cup ketchup
1 onion, diced	¼ cup sugar
15 ounces (425 g) canned garbanzo beans	1 teaspoon ground mustard powder
2 cups water	1 teaspoon salt
1 cup apple cider	1 teaspoon black pepper
2 garlic cloves, minced	Fresh parsley, for garnish

1. Cook pancetta for 5 minutes, until crispy, on Sauté mode. Add onion and garlic, and cook for 3 minutes until soft. Mix in garbanzo beans, ketchup, sugar, salt, apple cider, mustard powder, water, and pepper.
2. Seal the lid, press Bean/Chili and cook on High Pressure for 30 minutes. Release pressure naturally for 10 minutes. Serve in bowls garnished with parsley.

Per Serving

calories: 163 | fat: 5.7g | protein: 5.4g | carbs: 22.1g | fiber: 3.7g | sodium: 705mg

Brown Rice Stuffed Portobello Mushrooms

Prep time: 15 minutes | Cook time: 10 minutes | Serves 4

4 large portobello mushrooms, stems and gills removed

2 tablespoons olive oil

½ cup brown rice, cooked

1 tomato, seed removed and chopped

¼ cup black olives, pitted and chopped

1 green bell pepper, seeded and diced

½ cup feta cheese, crumbled

Juice of 1 lemon

½ teaspoon salt

½ teaspoon ground black pepper

Minced fresh cilantro, for garnish

1 cup vegetable broth

1. Brush the mushrooms with olive oil. Arrange the mushrooms in a single layer in an oiled baking pan. In a bowl, mix the rice, tomato, olives, bell pepper, feta cheese, lemon juice, salt, and black pepper.

2. Spoon the rice mixture into the mushrooms. Pour in the broth, seal the lid and cook on High Pressure for 10 minutes. Do a quick release. Garnish with fresh cilantro and serve immediately.

Per Serving

calories: 190 | fat: 12.5g | protein: 5.9g | carbs: 15.2g | fiber: 2.6g | sodium: 682mg

Sauces, Dips, and Dressings

Vinaigrette

Prep time: 5 minutes | Cook time: 0 minutes | Makes 1 cup

½ cup extra-virgin olive oil

¼ cup red wine vinegar

1 tablespoon Dijon mustard

1 teaspoon dried rosemary

½ teaspoon salt

½ teaspoon freshly ground black pepper

1. In a cup or a mansion jar with a lid, combine the olive oil, vinegar, mustard, rosemary, salt, and pepper and shake until well combined.
2. Serve chilled or at room temperature.

Per Serving

calories: 124 | fat: 14.0g | protein: 0g | carbs: 1.0g | fiber: 0g | sodium: 170mg

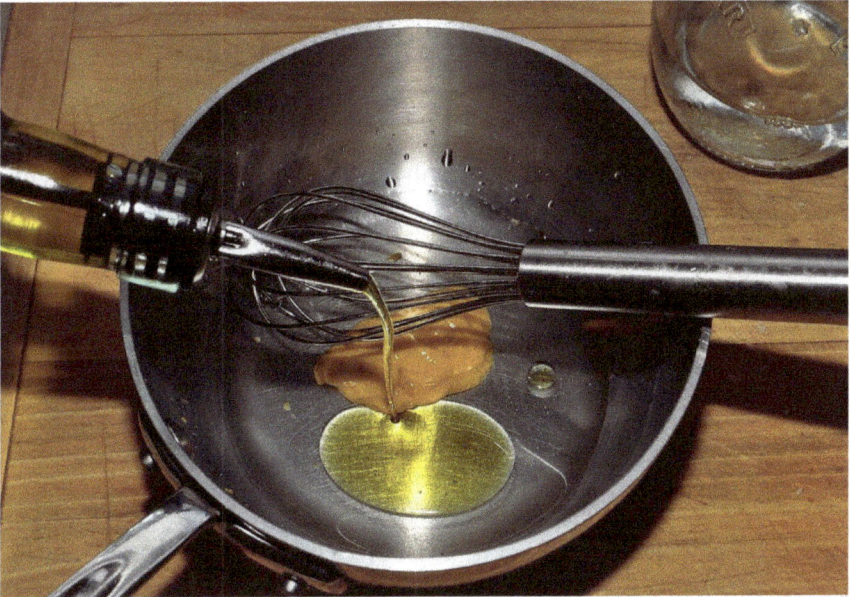

Ginger Teriyaki Sauce

Prep time: 5 minutes | Cook time: 0 minutes | Serves 2

¼ cup pineapple juice

¼ cup low-sodium soy sauce

2 tablespoons packed coconut sugar

1 tablespoon grated fresh ginger

1 tablespoon arrowroot powder or cornstarch

1 teaspoon garlic powder

1. Whisk the pineapple juice, soy sauce, coconut sugar, ginger, arrowroot powder, and garlic powder together in a small bowl.
2. Store in an airtight container in the fridge for up to 5 days.

Per Serving

calories: 37 | fat: 0.1g | protein: 1.1g | carbs: 12.0g | fiber: 0g | sodium: 881mg

Aioli

Prep time: 5 minutes | Cook time: 0 minutes | Makes ½ cup

½ cup plain Greek yogurt   ½ teaspoon hot sauce

2 teaspoons Dijon mustard   ¼ teaspoon raw honey

Pinch salt

1. In a small bowl, whisk together the yogurt, mustard, hot sauce, honey, and salt.
2. Serve immediately or refrigerate in an airtight container for up to 3 days.

Per Serving

calories: 47 | fat: 2.5g | protein: 2.1g | carbs: 3.5g | fiber: 0g | sodium: 231mg

Parsley Vinaigrette

Prep time: 5 minutes | Cook time: 0 minutes | Makes about ½ cup

½ cup lightly packed fresh parsley, finely chopped

⅓ cup extra-virgin olive oil

3 tablespoons red wine vinegar

1 garlic clove, minced

¼ teaspoon salt, plus additional as needed

1. Place all the ingredients in a mason jar and cover. Shake vigorously for 1 minute until completely mixed.
2. Taste and add additional salt as needed.
3. Serve immediately or serve chilled.

Per Serving (1 tablespoon)

calories: 92 | fat: 10.9g | protein: 0g | carbs: 0g | fiber: 0g | sodium: 75mg

Fish and Seafood

Hazelnut Crusted Sea Bass

Prep time: 10 minutes | Cook time: 15 minutes | Serves 2

2 tablespoons almond butter $\frac{1}{3}$ cup roasted hazelnuts

2 sea bass fillets   A pinch of cayenne pepper

1. Preheat the oven to 425ºF (220ºC). Line a baking dish with waxed paper.
2. Brush the almond butter over the fillets.
3. Pulse the hazelnuts and cayenne in a food processor. Coat the sea bass with the hazelnut mixture, then transfer to the baking dish.
4. Bake in the preheated oven for about 15 minutes. Cool for 5 minutes before serving.

Per Serving

calories: 468 | fat: 30.8g | protein: 40.0g | carbs: 8.8g | fiber: 4.1g | sodium: 90mg

Shrimp and Pea Paella

Prep time: 20 minutes | Cook time: 60 minutes | Serves 2

2 tablespoons olive oil

1 garlic clove, minced

½ large onion, minced

1 cup diced tomato

½ cup short-grain rice

½ teaspoon sweet paprika

½ cup dry white wine

1¼ cups low-sodium chicken stock

8 ounces (227 g) large raw shrimp'

1 cup frozen peas

¼ cup jarred roasted red peppers, cut into strips

Salt, to taste

1. Heat the olive oil in a large skillet over medium-high heat.
2. Add the garlic and onion and sauté for 3 minutes, or until the onion is softened.

3. Add the tomato, rice, and paprika and stir for 3 minutes to toast the rice.

4. Add the wine and chicken stock and stir to combine. Bring the mixture to a boil.

5. Cover and reduce the heat to medium-low, and simmer for 45 minutes, or until the rice is just about tender and most of the liquid has been absorbed.

6. Add the shrimp, peas, and roasted red peppers. Cover and cook for an additional 5 minutes. Season with salt to taste and serve.

Per Serving

calories: 646 | fat: 27.1g | protein: 42.0g | carbs: 59.7g | fiber: 7.0g | sodium: 687mg

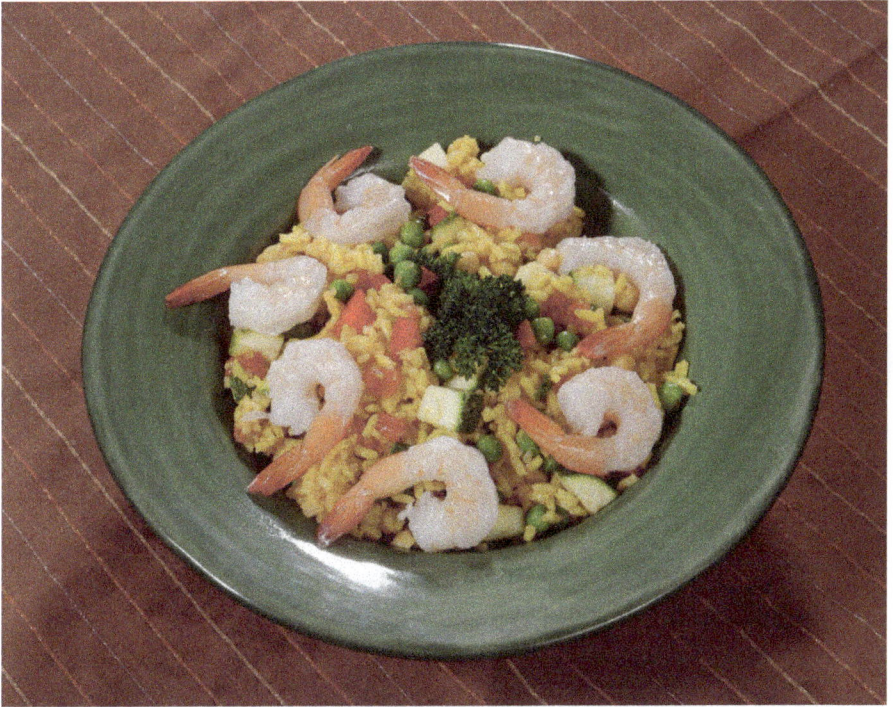

Garlic Shrimp with Arugula Pesto

Prep time: 20 minutes | Cook time: 5 minutes | Serves 2

3 cups lightly packed arugula

½ cup lightly packed basil leaves

¼ cup walnuts

3 tablespoons olive oil

3 medium garlic cloves

2 tablespoons grated Parmesan cheese

1 tablespoon freshly squeezed lemon juice

Salt and freshly ground black pepper, to taste

1 (10-ounce / 283-g) package zucchini noodles

8 ounces (227 g) cooked, shelled shrimp

2 Roma tomatoes, diced

1. Process the arugula, basil, walnuts, olive oil, garlic, Parmesan cheese, and lemon juice in a food processor until smooth, scraping down the sides as needed. Season with salt and pepper to taste.

2. Heat a skillet over medium heat. Add the pesto, zucchini noodles, and cooked shrimp. Toss to

combine the sauce over the noodles and shrimp, and cook until heated through.

3. Taste and season with more salt and pepper as needed. Serve topped with the diced tomatoes.

Per Serving

calories: 435 | fat: 30.2g | protein: 33.0g | carbs: 15.1g | fiber: 5.0g | sodium: 413mg

Lemony Salmon

Prep time: 10 minutes | Cook time: 3 minutes | Serves 3

1 cup water	1 teaspoon fresh lemon
3 lemon slices	juice
1 (5-ounce / 142-g)	Salt and ground black
salmon fillet	pepper, to taste
	Fresh cilantro to garnish

1. Add the water to the Instant pot and place a trivet inside.
2. In a shallow bowl, place the salmon fillet. Sprinkle salt and pepper over it.
3. Squeeze some lemon juice on top then place a lemon slice over the salmon fillet.
4. Cover the lid and lock it. Set its pressure release handle to Sealing position.
5. Use Steam function on your cooker for 3 minutes to cook.
6. After the beep, do a Quick release and release the pressure.
7. Remove the lid, then serve with the lemon slice and fresh cilantro on top.

Per Serving

calories: 161 | fat: 5.0g | protein: 26.6g | carbs: 0.7g | fiber: 0.2g | sodium: 119mg

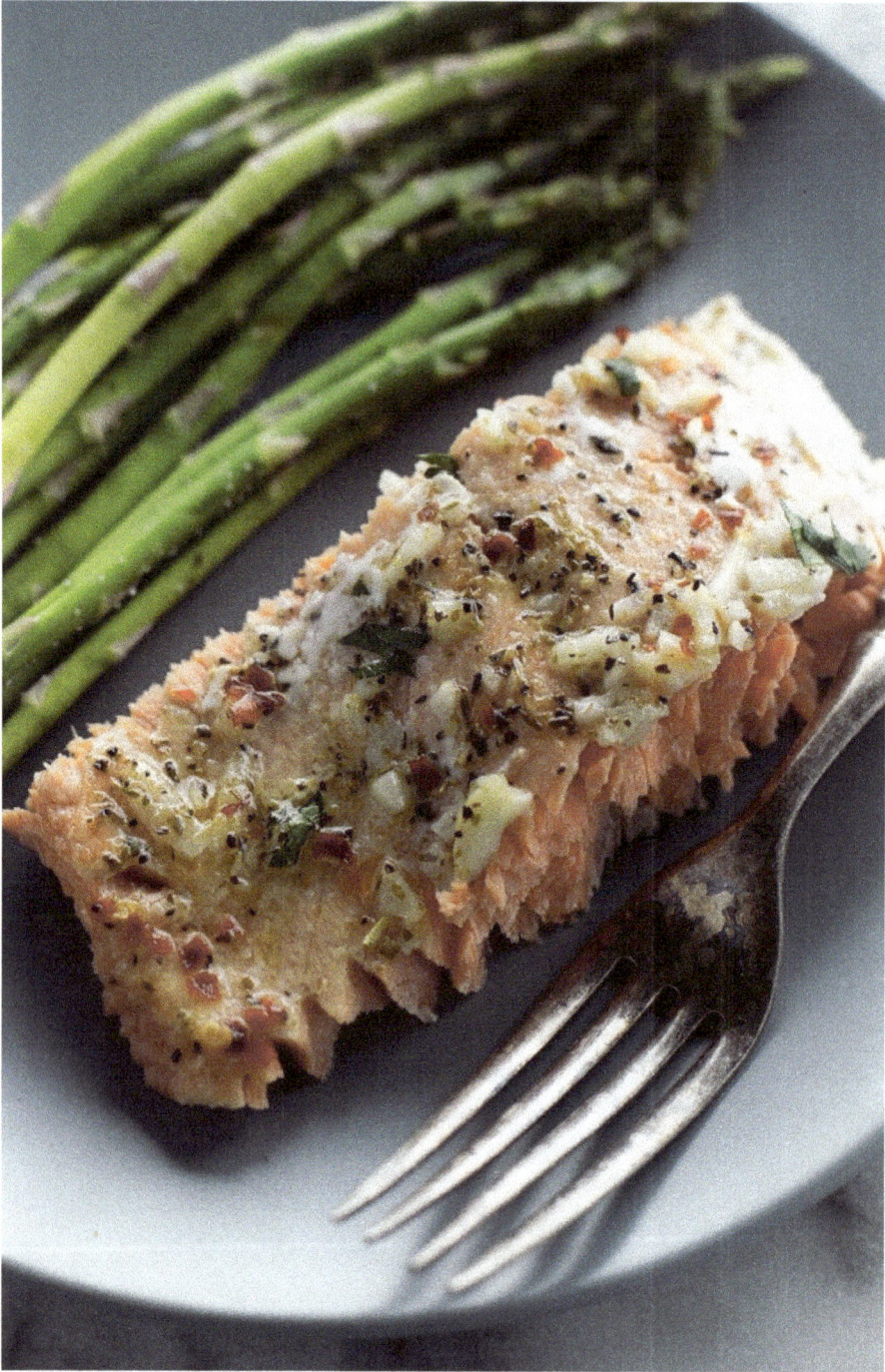

Spicy Cumin Salmon

Prep time: 10 minutes | Cook time: 2 minutes | Serves 8

2 cups water

2 garlic cloves, minced

2 teaspoons powdered stevia

8 lemon slices

2 tablespoons red chili powder

2 teaspoons ground cumin

Salt and freshly grated black pepper, to taste

2 pounds (907 g) salmon fillet, cut into 8 pieces

1. Pour two cups of water in the insert of the Instant Pot. Set the trivet in it.
2. In a separate bowl, add all the ingredients except the lemon slices and mix them well.
3. Pour this mixture over the salmon fillets and rub it all over it.
4. Place the salmon slices over the trivet in a single layer.
5. Top each fillet with a lemon slice.
6. Secure the lid and select Steam function for 2 minutes.

7. After the beep, do a Quick release and then remove the lid.

8. Serve immediately.

Per Serving

calories: 151 | fat: 4.7g | protein: 23.3g | carbs: 3.1g | fiber: 1.0g | sodium: 117mg

Rosemary Salmon with Feta Cheese

Prep time: 5 minutes | Cook time: 3 minutes | Serves 6

1½ pounds (680 g) salmon fillets

1½ cups water

¼ cup olive oil

1½ garlic cloves, minced

1½ tablespoons feta cheese, crumbled

½ teaspoon dried oregano

3 tablespoons fresh lemon juice

Salt and freshly ground black pepper, to taste

3 fresh rosemary sprigs

3 lemon slices

1. Take a large bowl and add the garlic, feta cheese, salt, pepper, lemon juice, and oregano. Whisk well all the ingredients.
2. Add the water to the Instant pot then place the steamer trivet in it.
3. Arrange the salmon fillets over the trivet in a single layer.
4. Pour the cheese mixture over these fillets.
5. Place a lemon slice and a rosemary sprig over each fillet.

6. Secure the lid.

7. Select the Steam function on your cooker and set 3 minutes cooking time.

8. After it is done, carefully do a Quick release. Remove the lid.

9. Serve hot.

Per Serving

calories: 229 | fat: 14.0g | protein: 23.4g | carbs: 1.3g | fiber: 0.2g | sodium: 88mg

Mahi-Mahi Meal

Prep time: 15 minutes | Cook time: 7 minutes | Serves 4

1½ cups water

4 (4-ounce / 113-g) mahi-mahi fillets

Salt and freshly ground black pepper, to taste

4 garlic cloves, minced

4 tablespoons fresh lime juice

4 tablespoons erythritol

2 teaspoons red pepper flakes, crushed

1. Sprinkle some salt and pepper over Mahi-Mahi fillets for seasoning.
2. In a separate bowl add all the remaining ingredients and mix well.
3. Add the water to the Instant pot and place the trivet in it.
4. Arrange the seasoned fillets over the trivet in a single layer.
5. Pour the prepared sauce on top of each fillet.
6. Cover and secure the lid.
7. Set the Steam function on your cooker for 5 minutes.

8. Once it beeps, do a quick release then remove the lid.

9. Serve the steaming hot Mahi-Mahi and enjoy.

Per Serving

calories: 228 | fat: 1.4g | protein: 38.0g | carbs: 14.2g | fiber: 0.1g | sodium: 182mg

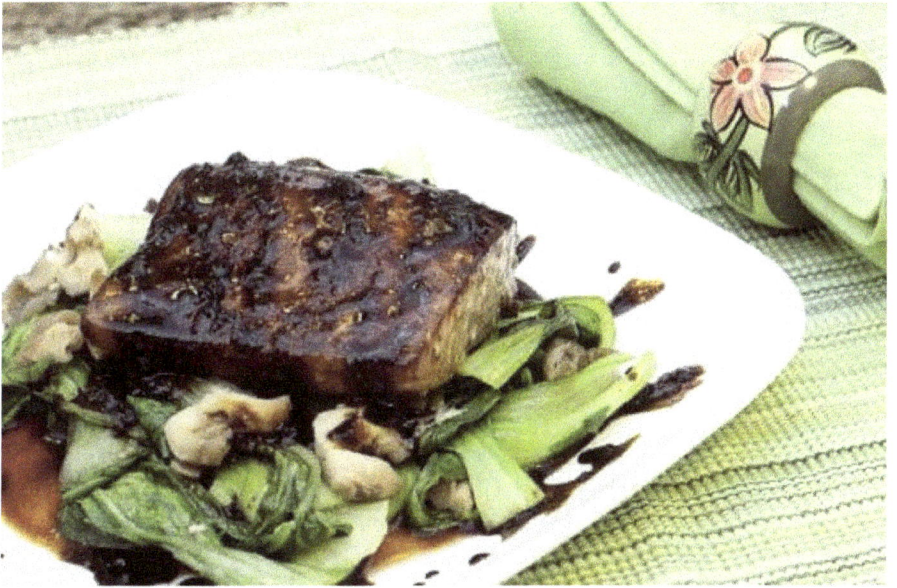

Rosemary Cod with Cherry Tomato

Prep time: 20 minutes | Cook time: 5 minutes | Serves 6

1½ pounds (680 g) cherry tomatoes, halved

2½ tablespoons fresh rosemary, chopped

6 (4-ounce / 113-g) cod fillets

3 garlic cloves, minced

2 tablespoons olive oil

Salt and freshly ground black pepper, to taste

1. Add the olive oil, half of the tomatoes and rosemary to the insert of the Instant Pot.
2. Place the cod fillets over these tomatoes. Then add more tomatoes to the pot.
3. Add the garlic to the pot. Then secure the lid.
4. Select the Manual function with High Pressure for 5 minutes.
5. After the beep, use the quick release to discharge all the steam.
6. Serve cod fillets with tomatoes and sprinkle a pinch of salt and pepper on top.

Per Serving

calories: 143 | fat: 5.2g | protein: 18.8g | carbs: 5.0g | fiber: 1.5g | sodium: 358mg

Baked Oysters with Vegetables

Prep time: 30 minutes | Cook time: 15 to 17 minutes | Serves 2

2 cups coarse salt, for holding the oysters

1 dozen fresh oysters, scrubbed

1 tablespoon almond butter

¼ cup finely chopped scallions, both white and green parts

½ cup finely chopped artichoke hearts

¼ cup finely chopped red bell pepper

1 garlic clove, minced

1 tablespoon finely chopped fresh parsley

Zest and juice of ½ lemon

Pinch salt

Freshly ground black pepper, to taste

1. Pour the salt into a baking dish and spread to evenly fill the bottom of the dish.
2. Prepare a clean work surface to shuck the oysters. Using a shucking knife, insert the blade

at the joint of the shell, where it hinges open and shut. Firmly apply pressure to pop the blade in, and work the knife around the shell to open. Discard the empty half of the shell. Using the knife, gently loosen the oyster, and remove any shell particles. Set the oysters in their shells on the salt, being careful not to spill the juices.

3. Preheat the oven to 425ºF (220ºC).

4. Heat the almond butter in a large skillet over medium heat. Add the scallions, artichoke hearts, and bell pepper, and cook for 5 to 7 minutes. Add the garlic and cook for 1 minute more.

5. Remove from the heat and stir in the parsley, lemon zest and juice, and season to taste with salt and pepper.

6. Divide the vegetable mixture evenly among the oysters. Bake in the preheated oven for 10 to 12 minutes, or until the vegetables are lightly browned. Serve warm.

Per Serving

calories: 135 | fat: 7.2g | protein: 6.0g | carbs: 10.7g | fiber: 2.0g | sodium: 280mg

Steamed Cod

Prep time: 15 minutes | Cook time: 7 minutes | Serves 4

1 pound (454 g) cherry tomatoes, halved	2 cups water
1 bunch fresh thyme sprigs	1 cup white rice
4 fillets cod	1 cup Kalamata olives
1 teaspoon olive oil	2 tablespoons pickled capers
1 clove garlic, pressed	1 tablespoon olive oil
3 pinches salt	1 pinch ground black pepper

1. Line a parchment paper on the basket of your instant pot. Place about half the tomatoes in a single layer on the paper. Sprinkle with thyme, reserving some for garnish.
2. Arrange cod fillets on top. Sprinkle with a little bit of olive oil.
3. Spread the garlic, pepper, salt, and remaining tomatoes over the fish. In the pot, mix rice and water.
4. Lay a trivet over the rice and water. Lower steamer basket onto the trivet.

5. Seal the lid, and cook for 7 minutes on Low Pressure. Release the pressure quickly.

6. Remove the steamer basket and trivet from the pot. Use a fork to fluff rice.

7. Plate the fish fillets and apply a garnish of olives, reserved thyme, pepper, remaining olive oil, and capers. Serve with rice.

Per Serving

calories: 352 | fat: 9.1g | protein: 22.2g | carbs: 44.7g | fiber: 3.9g | sodium: 827mg

Steamed Bass

Prep time: 10 minutes | Cook time: 8 minutes | Serves 4

1½ cups water

1 lemon, sliced

4 sea bass fillets

4 sprigs thyme

1 white onion, cut into thin rings

2 turnips, chopped

2 pinches salt

1 pinch ground black pepper

2 teaspoons olive oil

1. Add water and set a rack into the pot.
2. Line a parchment paper to the bottom of the steamer basket. Place lemon slices in a single layer on the rack.
3. Arrange fillets on the top of the lemons, cover with onion and thyme sprigs. Top with turnip slices.
4. Drizzle pepper, salt, and olive oil over the mixture. Put steamer basket onto the rack.
5. Seal lid and cook on Low pressure for 8 minutes. Release the pressure quickly.

6. Serve over the delicate onion rings and thinly turnips.

Per Serving

calories: 177 | fat: 4.9g | protein: 24.7g | carbs: 7.8g | fiber: 2.0g | sodium: 209mg

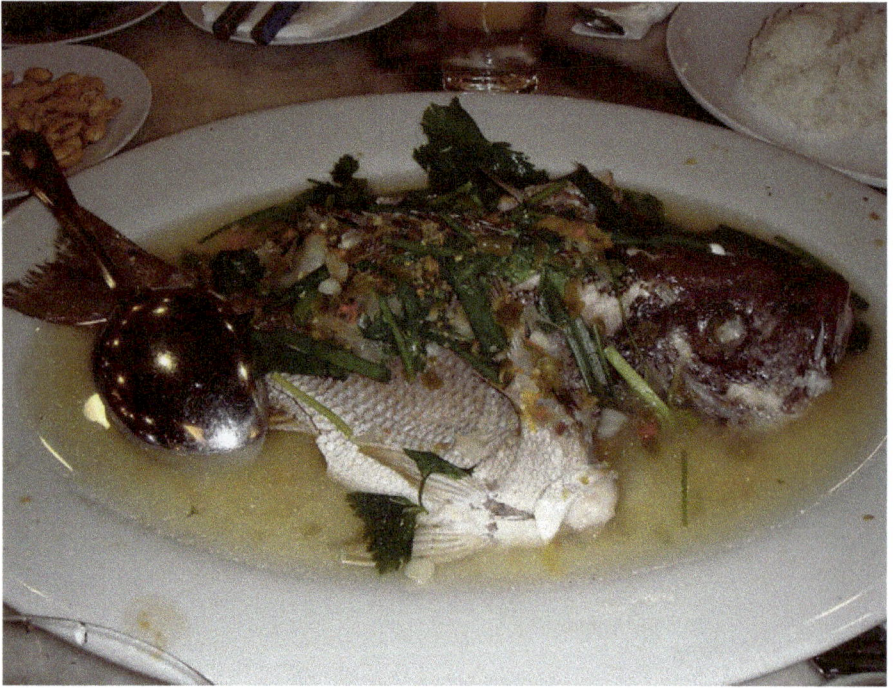

Catfish and Shrimp Jambalaya

Prep time: 20 minutes | Cook time: 4 hours 45 minutes | Serves

4 ounces (113 g) catfish (cut into 1-inch cubes)

4 ounces (113 g) shrimp (peeled and deveined)

1 tablespoon olive oil

2 bacon slices, chopped

1¼ cups vegetable broth

¾ cup sliced celery stalk

¼ teaspoon minced garlic

½ cup chopped onion

1 cup canned diced tomatoes

1 cup uncooked long-grain white rice

½ tablespoon Cajun seasoning

¼ teaspoon dried thyme

¼ teaspoon cayenne pepper

½ teaspoon dried oregano

Salt and freshly ground black pepper, to taste

1. Select the Sauté function on your Instant Pot and add the oil into it.
2. Put the onion, garlic, celery, and bacon to the pot and cook for 10 minutes.

3. Add all the remaining ingredients to the pot except seafood.

4. Stir well, then secure the cooker lid.

5. Select the Slow Cook function on a medium mode.

6. Keep the pressure release handle on venting position. Cook for 4 hours.

7. Once done, remove the lid and add the seafood to the gravy.

8. Secure the lid again, keep the pressure handle in the venting position.

9. Cook for another 45 minutes then serve.

Per Serving

calories: 437 | fat: 13.1g | protein: 21.3g | carbs: 56.7g | fiber: 2.6g | sodium: 502mg

Salmon and Potato Casserole

Prep time: 20 minutes | Cook time: 8 hours | Serves 4

½ tablespoon olive oil

8 ounces (227 g) cream of mushroom soup

¼ cup water

3 medium potatoes (peeled and sliced)

3 tablespoons flour

1 (1-pound / 454-g) can salmon (drained and flaked)

½ cup chopped scallion

¼ teaspoon ground nutmeg

Salt and freshly ground black pepper, to taste

1. Pour mushroom soup and water in a separate bowl and mix them well.
2. Add the olive oil to the Instant Pot and grease it lightly.
3. Place half of the potatoes in the pot and sprinkle salt, pepper, and half of the flour over it.
4. Now add a layer of half of the salmon over potatoes, then a layer of half of the scallions.
5. Repeat these layers and pour mushroom soup mix on top.
6. Top it with nutmeg evenly.

7. Secure the lid and set its pressure release handle to the venting position.

8. Select the Slow Cook function with Medium heat on your Instant Pot.

9. Let it cook for 8 hours then serve.

Per Serving

calories: 388 | fat: 11.6g | protein: 34.6g | carbs: 37.2g | fiber: 4.4g | sodium: 842mg

Salmon and Tomato Curry

Prep time: 10 minutes | Cook time: 12 minutes | Serves 8

3 pounds (1.4 kg) salmon fillets (cut into pieces)

2 tablespoons olive oil

2 Serrano peppers, chopped

1 teaspoon ground turmeric

4 tablespoons curry powder

4 teaspoons ground cumin

4 curry leaves

4 teaspoons ground coriander

2 small yellow onions, chopped

2 teaspoons red chili powder

4 garlic cloves, minced

4 cups unsweetened coconut milk

2½ cups tomatoes, chopped

2 tablespoons fresh lemon juice

Fresh cilantro leaves to garnish

1. Put the oil and curry leaves to the insert of the Instant Pot. Select the Sauté function to cook for 30 secs.

2. Add the garlic and onions to the pot, cook for 5 minutes.
3. Stir in all the spices and cook for another 1 minute.
4. Put the fish, Serrano pepper, coconut milk, and tomatoes while cooking.
5. Cover and lock the lid. Seal the pressure release valve.
6. Select the Manual function at Low Pressure for 5 minutes.
7. After the beep, do a Natural release to release all the steam.
8. Remove the lid and squeeze in lemon juice.
9. Garnish with fresh cilantro leaves and serve.

Per Serving

calories: 551 | fat: 40.6g | protein: 38.9g | carbs: 10.6g | fiber: 3.2g | sodium: 778mg

Fruits and Desserts

Rice Pudding with Roasted Orange

Prep time: 10 minutes | Cook time: 19 to 20 minutes | Serves 6

2 medium oranges

2 teaspoons extra-virgin olive oil

⅛ teaspoon kosher salt

2 large eggs

2 cups unsweetened almond milk

1 cup orange juice

1 cup uncooked instant brown rice

¼ cup honey

½ teaspoon ground cinnamon

1 teaspoon vanilla extract

Cooking spray

1. Preheat the oven to 450ºF (235ºC). Spritz a large, rimmed baking sheet with cooking spray. Set aside.

2. Slice the unpeeled oranges into ¼-inch rounds. Brush with the oil and sprinkle with salt. Place the slices on the baking sheet and roast for 4

minutes. Flip the slices and roast for 4 more minutes, or until they begin to brown. Remove from the oven and set aside.

3. Crack the eggs into a medium bowl. In a medium saucepan, whisk together the milk, orange juice, rice, honey and cinnamon. Bring to a boil over medium-high heat, stirring constantly. Reduce the heat to medium- low and simmer for 10 minutes, stirring occasionally.

4. Using a measuring cup, scoop out ½ cup of the hot rice mixture and whisk it into the eggs. While constantly stirring the mixture in the pan, slowly pour the egg mixture back into the saucepan. Cook on low heat for 1 to 2 minutes, or until thickened, stirring constantly. Remove from the heat and stir in the vanilla.

5. Let the pudding stand for a few minutes for the rice to soften. The rice will be cooked but slightly chewy. For softer rice, let stand for another half hour.

6. Top with the roasted oranges. Serve warm or at room temperature.

Per Serving

calories: 204 | fat: 6.0g | protein: 5.0g | carbs: 34.0g |
fiber: 1.0g | sodium: 148mg

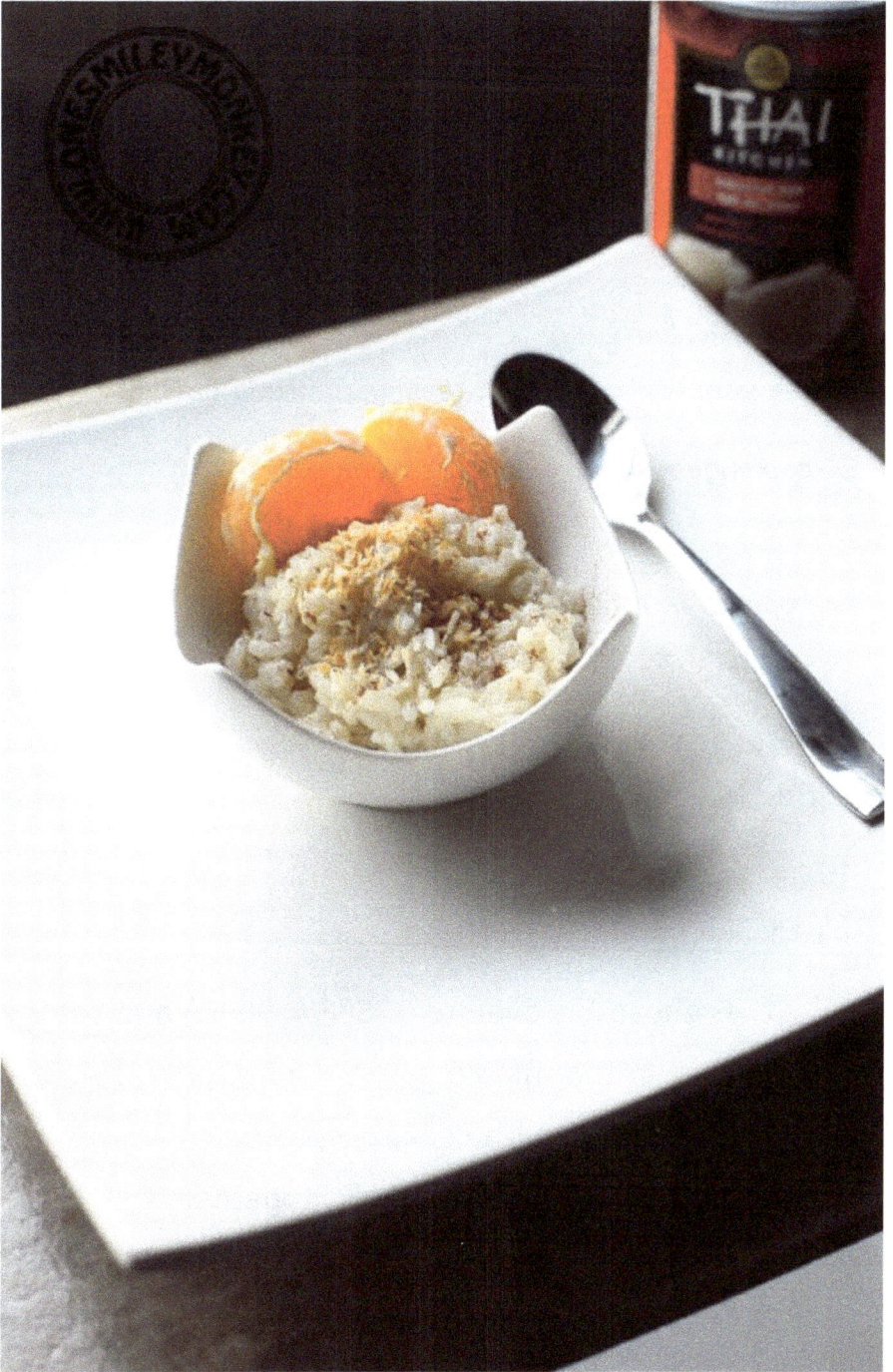

Cherry Walnut Brownies

Prep time: 10 minutes | Cook time: 20 minutes | Serves 9

2 large eggs

½ cup 2% plain Greek yogurt

½ cup sugar 1⁄3 cup honey

¼ cup extra-virgin olive oil

1 teaspoon vanilla extract

½ cup whole-wheat pastry flour

1⁄3 cup unsweetened dark chocolate cocoa powder

¼ teaspoon baking powder

¼ teaspoon salt

1⁄3 cup chopped walnuts

9 fresh cherries, stemmed and pitted

Cooking spray

1. Preheat the oven to 375ºF (190ºC) and set the rack in the middle of the oven. Spritz a square baking pan with cooking spray.
2. In a large bowl, whisk together the eggs, yogurt, sugar, honey, oil and vanilla.
3. In a medium bowl, stir together the flour, cocoa powder, baking powder and salt. Add the flour

mixture to the egg mixture and whisk until all the dry ingredients are incorporated. Fold in the walnuts.

4. Pour the batter into the prepared pan. Push the cherries into the batter, three to a row in three rows, so one will be at the center of each brownie once you cut them into squares.

5. Bake the brownies for 20 minutes, or until just set. Remove from the oven and place on a rack to cool for 5 minutes. Cut into nine squares and serve.

Per Serving

calories: 154 | fat: 6.0g | protein: 3.0g | carbs: 24.0g | fiber: 2.0g | sodium: 125mg

Watermelon and Blueberry Salad

Prep time: 5 minutes | Cook time: 0 minutes | Serves 6 to 8

1 medium watermelon

1 cup fresh blueberries

1⁄ cup honey

2 tablespoons lemon juice

2 tablespoons finely chopped fresh mint leaves

1. Cut the watermelon into 1-inch cubes. Put them in a bowl.
2. Evenly distribute the blueberries over the watermelon.
3. In a separate bowl, whisk together the honey, lemon juice and mint.
4. Drizzle the mint dressing over the watermelon and blueberries.
5. Serve cold.

Per Serving

calories: 238 | fat: 1.0g | protein: 4.0g | carbs: 61.0g | fiber: 3.0g | sodium: 11mg

Crispy Sesame Cookies

Prep time: 5 minutes | Cook time: 8 to 10 minutes | Serves 14 to 16

1 cup hulled sesame seeds   8 tablespoons almond butter

1 cup sugar   2 large eggs

                            1¼ cups flour

1. Preheat the oven to 350ºF (180ºC).
2. Toast the sesame seeds on a baking sheet for 3 minutes. Set aside and let cool.
3. Using a mixer, whisk together the sugar and butter. Add the eggs one at a time until well blended. Add the flour and toasted sesame seeds and mix until well blended.
4. Drop spoonfuls of cookie dough onto a baking sheet and form them into round balls, about 1-inch in diameter, similar to a walnut.
5. Put in the oven and bake for 5 to 7 minutes, or until golden brown.
6. Let the cookies cool for 5 minutes before serving.

Per Serving

calories: 218 | fat: 12.0g | protein: 4.0g | carbs: 25.0g | fiber: 2.0g | sodium: 58mg

Mint Banana Chocolate Sorbet

Prep time: 4 hours 5 minutes | Cook time: 0 minutes | Serves 1

1 frozen banana

1 tablespoon almond butter

2 tablespoons minced fresh mint

2 to 3 tablespoons dark chocolate chips (60% cocoa or higher)

2 to 3 tablespoons goji (optional)

1. Put the banana, butter, and mint in a food processor. Pulse to purée until creamy and smooth.
2. Add the chocolate and goji, then pulse for several more times to combine well.
3. Pour the mixture in a bowl or a ramekin, then freeze for at least 4 hours before serving chilled.

Per Serving

calories: 213 | fat: 9.8g | protein: 3.1g | carbs: 2.9g | fiber: 4.0g | sodium: 155mg

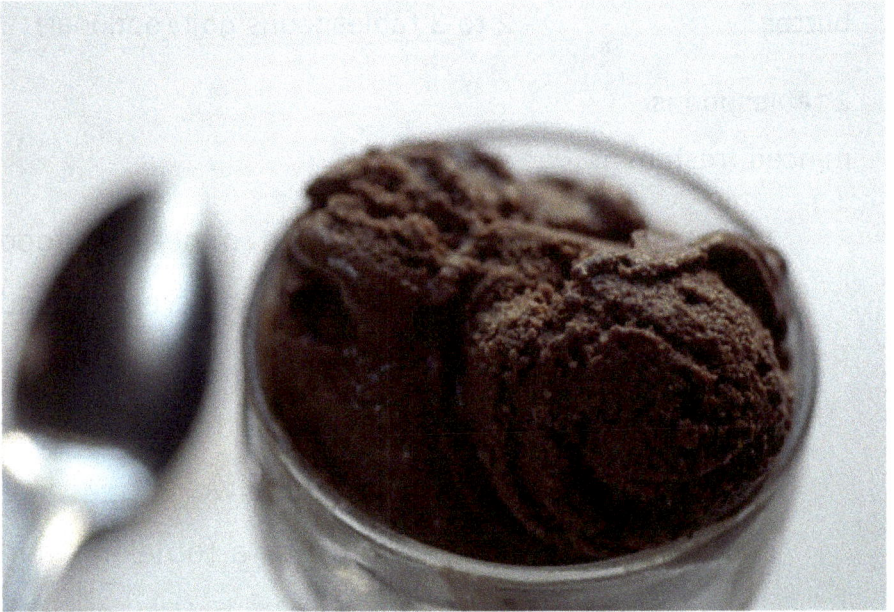

Pecan and Carrot Cake

Prep time: 15 minutes | Cook time: 45 minutes | Serves 12

½ cup coconut oil, at room temperature, plus more for greasing the baking dish

2 teaspoons pure vanilla extract

¼ cup pure maple syrup 6 eggs

½ cup coconut flour

1 teaspoon baking powder

1 teaspoon baking soda

½ teaspoon ground nutmeg

1 teaspoon ground cinnamon

⅛ teaspoon sea salt

½ cup chopped pecans

3 cups finely grated carrots

1. Preheat the oven to 350ºF (180ºC). Grease a 13-by-9-inch baking dish with coconut oil.
2. Combine the vanilla extract, maple syrup, and ½ cup of coconut oil in a large bowl. Stir to mix well.

3. Break the eggs in the bowl and whisk to combine well. Set aside.

4. Combine the coconut flour, baking powder, baking soda, nutmeg, cinnamon, and salt in a separate bowl. Stir to mix well.

5. Make a well in the center of the flour mixture, then pour the egg mixture into the well. Stir to combine well.

6. Add the pecans and carrots to the bowl and toss to mix well. Pour the mixture in the single layer on the baking dish.

7. Bake in the preheated oven for 45 minutes or until puffed and the cake spring back when lightly press with your fingers.

8. Remove the cake from the oven. Allow to cool for at least 15 minutes, then serve.

Per Serving

calories: 255 | fat: 21.2g | protein: 5.1g | carbs: 12.8g | fiber: 2.0g | sodium: 202mg

Raspberry Yogurt Basted Cantaloupe

Prep time: 15 minutes | Cook time: 0 minutes | Serves 6

2 cups fresh raspberries, mashed

1 cup plain coconut yogurt

½ teaspoon vanilla extract

1 cantaloupe, peeled and sliced

½ cup toasted coconut flakes

1. Combine the mashed raspberries with yogurt and vanilla extract in a small bowl. Stir to mix well.
2. Place the cantaloupe slices on a platter, then top with raspberry mixture and spread with toasted coconut.
3. Serve immediately.

Per Serving

calories: 75 | fat: 4.1g | protein: 1.2g | carbs: 10.9g | fiber: 6.0g | sodium: 36mg

Apple Compote

Prep time: 15 minutes | Cook time: 10 minutes | Serves 4

6 apples, peeled, cored, and chopped

¼ cup raw honey

1 teaspoon ground cinnamon

¼ cup apple juice

Sea salt, to taste

1. Put all the ingredients in a stockpot. Stir to mix well, then cook over medium-high heat for 10 minutes or until the apples are glazed by honey and lightly saucy. Stir constantly.
2. Serve immediately.

Per Serving

calories: 246 | fat: 0.9g | protein: 1.2g | carbs: 66.3g | fiber: 9.0g | sodium: 62mg

Peanut Butter and Chocolate Balls

Prep time: 45 minutes | Cook time: 0 minutes | Serves 15 balls

¾ cup creamy peanut butter

¼ cup unsweetened cocoa powder

2 tablespoons softened almond butter

½ teaspoon vanilla extract

1¾ cups maple syrup

1. Line a baking sheet with parchment paper.
2. Combine all the ingredients in a bowl. Stir to mix well.
3. Divide the mixture into 15 parts and shape each part into a 1-inch ball.
4. Arrange the balls on the baking sheet and refrigerate for at least 30 minutes, then serve chilled.

Per Serving (1 ball)

calories: 146 | fat: 8.1g | protein: 4.2g | carbs: 16.9g | fiber: 1.0g | sodium: 70mg

Spiced Sweet Pecans

Prep time: 4 minutes | Cook time: 17 minutes | Serves 4

1 cup pecan halves

3 tablespoons almond butter

1 teaspoon ground cinnamon

½ teaspoon ground nutmeg

¼ cup raw honey

¼ teaspoon sea salt

1. Preheat the oven to 350ºF (180ºC). Line a baking sheet with parchment paper.
2. Combine all the ingredients in a bowl. Stir to mix well, then spread the mixture in the single layer on the baking sheet with a spatula.
3. Bake in the preheated oven for 16 minutes or until the pecan halves are well browned.
4. Serve immediately.

Per Serving

calories: 324 | fat: 29.8g | protein: 3.2g | carbs: 13.9g | fiber: 4.0g | sodium: 180mg

Greek Yogurt Affogato with Pistachios

Prep time: 5 minutes | Cook time: 0 minutes | Serves 4

24 ounces (680 g) vanilla Greek yogurt

2 teaspoons sugar

4 shots hot espresso

4 tablespoons chopped unsalted pistachios

4 tablespoons dark chocolate chips

1. Spoon the yogurt into four bowls or tall glasses.
2. Mix ½ teaspoon of sugar into each of the espresso shots.
3. Pour one shot of the hot espresso over each bowl of yogurt.
4. Top each bowl with 1 tablespoon of the pistachios and 1 tablespoon of the chocolate chips and serve.

Per Serving

calories: 190 | fat: 6.0g | protein: 20.0g | carbs: 14.0g | fiber: 1.0g | sodium: 99mg

Grilled Peaches with Whipped Ricotta

Prep time: 5 minutes | Cook time: 14 to 22 minutes | Serves 4

4 peaches, halved and pitted

2 teaspoons extra-virgin olive oil

¾ cup whole-milk Ricotta cheese

1 tablespoon honey

¼ teaspoon freshly grated nutmeg

4 sprigs mint

Cooking spray

1. Spritz a grill pan with cooking spray. Heat the grill pan to medium heat.
2. Place a large, empty bowl in the refrigerator to chill.
3. Brush the peaches all over with the oil. Place half of the peaches, cut-side down, on the grill pan and cook for 3 to 5 minutes, or until grill marks appear.
4. Using tongs, turn the peaches over. Cover the grill pan with aluminum foil and cook for 4 to 6 minutes, or until the peaches are easily pierced

with a sharp knife. Set aside to cool. Repeat with the remaining peaches.

5. Remove the bowl from the refrigerator and add the Ricotta. Using an electric beater, beat the Ricotta on high for 2 minutes. Add the honey and nutmeg and beat for 1 more minute.

6. Divide the cooled peaches among 4 serving bowls. Top with the Ricotta mixture and a sprig of mint and serve.

Per Serving

calories: 176 | fat: 8.0g | protein: 8.0g | carbs: 20.0g | fiber: 3.0g | sodium: 63mg

Honey Baked Cinnamon Apples

Prep time: 5 minutes | Cook time: 20 minutes | Serves 2

1 teaspoon extra-virgin olive oil

4 firm apples, peeled, cored, and sliced

½ teaspoon salt

1½ teaspoons ground cinnamon, divided

2 tablespoons unsweetened almond milk

2 tablespoons honey

1. Preheat the oven to 375ºF (190ºC). Coat a small casserole dish with the olive oil.

2. Toss the apple slices with the salt and ½ teaspoon of the cinnamon in a medium bowl. Spread the apples in the prepared casserole dish and bake in the preheated oven for 20 minutes.

3. Meanwhile, in a small saucepan, heat the milk, honey, and remaining 1 teaspoon of cinnamon over medium heat, stirring frequently.

4. When it reaches a simmer, remove the pan from the heat and cover to keep warm.

5. Divide the apple slices between 2 plates and pour the sauce over the apples. Serve warm.

Per Serving

calories: 310 | fat: 3.4g | protein: 1.7g | carbs: 68.5g | fiber: 12.6g | sodium: 593mg

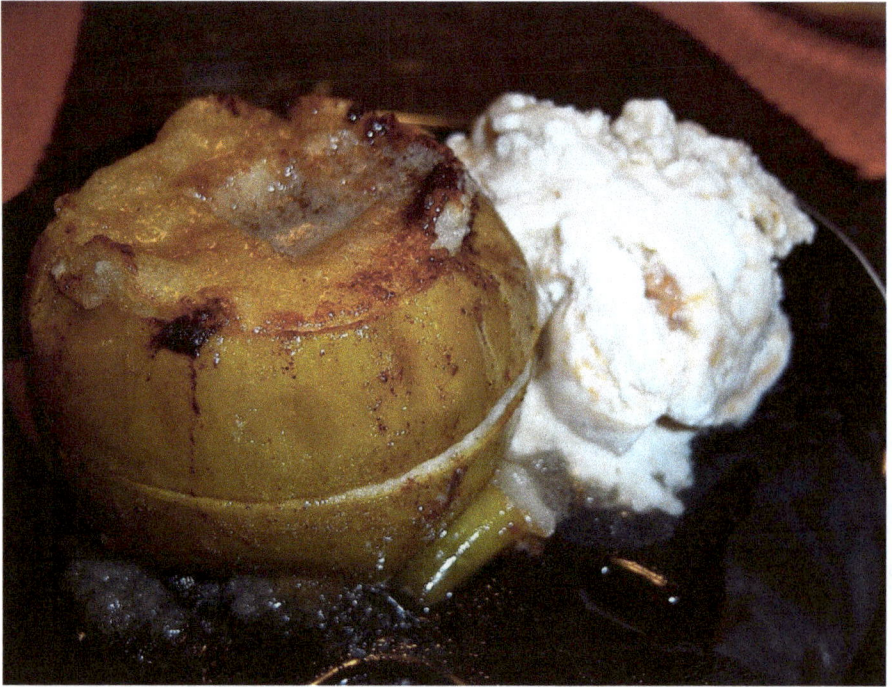

Strawberries with Balsamic Vinegar

Prep time: 5 minutes | Cook time: 0 minutes | Serves 2

2 cups strawberries, hulled and sliced

2 tablespoons sugar

2 tablespoons balsamic vinegar

1. Place the sliced strawberries in a bowl, sprinkle with the sugar, and drizzle lightly with the balsamic vinegar.
2. Toss to combine well and allow to sit for about 10 minutes before serving.

Per Serving

calories: 92 | fat: 0.4g | protein: 1.0g | carbs: 21.7g | fiber: 2.9g | sodium: 5mg

Frozen Mango Raspberry Delight

Prep time: 5 minutes | Cook time: 0 minutes | Serves 2

3 cups frozen raspberries   1 peach, peeled and pitted

1 mango, peeled and pitted   1 teaspoon honey

1. Place all the ingredients into a blender and purée, adding some water as needed.
2. Put in the freezer for 10 minutes to firm up if desired. Serve chilled or at room temperature.

Per Serving

calories: 276 | fat: 2.1g | protein: 4.5g | carbs: 60.3g | fiber: 17.5g | sodium: 4mg

Grilled Stone Fruit with Honey

Prep time: 8 minutes | Cook time: 6 minutes | Serves 2

3 apricots, halved and pitted

½ cup low-fat ricotta cheese

2 plums, halved and pitted

2 tablespoons honey

2 peaches, halved and pitted

Cooking spray

1. Preheat the grill to medium heat. Spray the grill grates with cooking spray.
2. Arrange the fruit, cut side down, on the grill, and cook for 2 to 3 minutes per side, or until lightly charred and softened.
3. Serve warm with a sprinkle of cheese and a drizzle of honey.

Per Serving

calories: 298 | fat: 7.8g | protein: 11.9g | carbs: 45.2g | fiber: 4.3g | sodium: 259mg

Mascarpone Baked Pears

Prep time: 10 minutes | Cook time: 20 minutes | Serves 2

2 ripe pears, peeled

1 tablespoon plus 2 teaspoons honey, divided

1 teaspoon vanilla, divided

¼ teaspoon ground coriander

¼ teaspoon ginger

¼ cup minced walnuts

¼ cup mascarpone cheese Pinch salt

Cooking spray

1. Preheat the oven to 350ºF (180ºC). Spray a small baking dish with cooking spray.
2. Slice the pears in half lengthwise. Using a spoon, scoop out the core from each piece. Put the pears, cut side up, in the baking dish.
3. Whisk together 1 tablespoon of honey, ½ teaspoon of vanilla, ginger, and coriander in a small bowl. Pour this mixture evenly over the pear halves.
4. Scatter the walnuts over the pear halves.
5. Bake in the preheated oven for 20 minutes, or until the pears are golden and you're able to pierce them easily with a knife.

6. Meanwhile, combine the mascarpone cheese with the remaining 2 teaspoons of honey, ½ teaspoon of vanilla, and a pinch of salt. Stir to combine well.

7. Divide the mascarpone among the warm pear halves and serve.

Per Serving

calories: 308 | fat: 16.0g | protein: 4.1g | carbs: 42.7g | fiber: 6.0g | sodium: 88mg

Mixed Berry Crisp

Prep time: 15 minutes | Cook time: 30 minutes | Serves 2

1½ cups frozen mixed berries, thawed

1 tablespoon coconut sugar

1 tablespoon almond butter

¼ cup oats

¼ cup pecans

1. Preheat the oven to 350ºF (180ºC).
2. Divide the mixed berries between 2 ramekins
3. Place the coconut sugar, almond butter, oats, and pecans in a food processor, and pulse a few times, until the mixture resembles damp sand.
4. Divide the crumble topping over the mixed berries.
5. Put the ramekins on a sheet pan and bake for 30 minutes, or until the top is golden and the berries are bubbling.
6. Serve warm.

Per Serving

calories: 268 | fat: 17.0g | protein: 4.1g | carbs: 26.8g | fiber: 6.0g | sodium: 44mg

Orange Mug Cakes

Prep time: 10 minutes | Cook time: 3 minutes | Serves 2

6 tablespoons flour

2 tablespoons sugar

1 teaspoon orange zest

½ teaspoon baking powder

Pinch salt

1 egg

2 tablespoons olive oil

2 tablespoons unsweetened almond milk

2 tablespoons freshly squeezed orange juice

½ teaspoon orange extract

½ teaspoon vanilla extract

1. Combine the flour, sugar, orange zest, baking powder, and salt in a small bowl.
2. In another bowl, whisk together the egg, olive oil, milk, orange juice, orange extract, and vanilla extract.
3. Add the dry ingredients to the wet ingredients and stir to incorporate. The batter will be thick.
4. Divide the mixture into two small mugs. Microwave each mug separately. The small ones should take about 60 seconds, and one

large mug should take about 90 seconds, but microwaves can vary.

5. Cool for 5 minutes before serving.

Per Serving

calories: 303 | fat: 16.9g | protein: 6.0g | carbs: 32.5g | fiber: 1.0g | sodium: 118mg

Fruit and Nut Chocolate Bark

Prep time: 15 minutes | Cook time: 2 minutes | Serves 2

2 tablespoons chopped nuts

3 ounces (85 g) dark chocolate chips

¼ cup chopped dried fruit (blueberries, apricots, figs, prunes, or any combination of those)

1. Line a sheet pan with parchment paper and set aside.
2. Add the nuts to a skillet over medium-high heat and toast for 60 seconds, or just fragrant. Set aside to cool.
3. Put the chocolate chips in a microwave-safe glass bowl and microwave on High for 1 minute.
4. Stir the chocolate and allow any unmelted chips to warm and melt. If desired, heat for an additional 20 to 30 seconds.
5. Transfer the chocolate to the prepared sheet pan. Scatter the dried fruit and toasted nuts over the chocolate evenly and gently pat in so they stick.

6. Place the sheet pan in the refrigerator for at least 1 hour to let the chocolate harden.

7. When ready, break into pieces and serve.

Per Serving

calories: 285 | fat: 16.1g | protein: 4.0g | carbs: 38.7g | fiber: 2.0g | sodium: 2mg

Crunchy Almond Cookies

Prep time: 5 minutes | Cook time: 5 to 7 minutes | Serves 4 to 6

½ cup sugar

1½ cups all-purpose flour

8 tablespoons almond butter

1 cup ground almonds

1 large egg

1. Preheat the oven to 375ºF (190ºC). Line a baking sheet with parchment paper.
2. Using a mixer, whisk together the sugar and butter. Add the egg and mix until combined. Alternately add the flour and ground almonds, ½ cup at a time, while the mixer is on slow.
3. Drop 1 tablespoon of the dough on the prepared baking sheet, keeping the cookies at least 2 inches apart.
4. Put the baking sheet in the oven and bake for about 5 to 7 minutes, or until the cookies start to turn brown around the edges.
5. Let cool for 5 minutes before serving.

Per Serving

calories: 604 | fat: 36.0g | protein: 11.0g | carbs: 63.0g | fiber: 4.0g | sodium: 181mg

Walnut and Date Balls

Prep time: 5 minutes | Cook time: 8 to 10 minutes | Serves 6 to 8

1 cup walnuts

1 cup unsweetened shredded coconut

14 medjool dates, pitted

8 tablespoons almond butter

1. Preheat the oven to 350ºF (180ºC).
2. Put the walnuts on a baking sheet and toast in the oven for 5 minutes.
3. Put the shredded coconut on a clean baking sheet. Toast for about 3 to 5 minutes, or until it turns golden brown. Once done, remove it from the oven and put it in a shallow bowl.
4. In a food processor, process the toasted walnuts until they have a medium chop. Transfer the chopped walnuts into a medium bowl.
5. Add the dates and butter to the food processor and blend until the dates become a thick paste. Pour the chopped walnuts into the food

processor with the dates and pulse just until the mixture is combined, about 5 to 7 pulses.

6. Remove the mixture from the food processor and scrape it into a large bowl.

7. To make the balls, spoon 1 to 2 tablespoons of the date mixture into the palm of your hand and roll around between your hands until you form a ball. Put the ball on a clean, lined baking sheet. Repeat until all the mixture is formed into balls.

8. Roll each ball in the toasted coconut until the outside of the ball is coated. Put the ball back on the baking sheet and repeat.

9. Put all the balls into the refrigerator for 20 minutes before serving. Store any leftovers in the refrigerator in an airtight container.

Per Serving

calories: 489 | fat: 35.0g | protein: 5.0g | carbs: 48.0g | fiber: 7.0g | sodium: 114mg

Apple and Berries Ambrosia

Prep time: 15 minutes | Cook time: 0 minutes | Serves 4

2 cups unsweetened coconut milk, chilled

2 tablespoons raw honey

1 apple, peeled, cored, and chopped

2 cups fresh raspberries

2 cups fresh blueberries

1. Spoon the chilled milk in a large bowl, then mix in the honey. Stir to mix well.
2. Then mix in the remaining ingredients. Stir to coat the fruits well and serve immediately.

Per Serving

calories: 386 | fat: 21.1g | protein: 4.2g | carbs: 45.9g | fiber: 11.0g | sodium: 16mg

Banana, Cranberry, and Oat Bars

Prep time: 15 minutes | Cook time: 40 minutes | Makes 16 bars

2 tablespoon extra-virgin olive oil

2 medium ripe bananas, mashed

½ cup almond butter

½ cup maple syrup

1⅓ cup dried cranberries

1½ cups old-fashioned rolled oats

¼ cup oat flour

¼ cup ground flaxseed

¼ teaspoon ground cloves

½ cup shredded coconut

½ teaspoon ground cinnamon

1 teaspoon vanilla extract

1. Preheat the oven to 400ºF (205ºC). Line a 8-inch square pan with parchment paper, then grease with olive oil.
2. Combine the mashed bananas, almond butter, and maple syrup in a bowl. Stir to mix well.
3. Mix in the remaining ingredients and stir to mix well until thick and sticky.
4. Spread the mixture evenly on the square pan with a spatula, then bake in the preheated oven

for 40 minutes or until a toothpick inserted in the center comes out clean.

5. Remove them from the oven and slice into 16 bars to serve.

Per Serving

calories: 145 | fat: 7.2g | protein: 3.1g | carbs: 18.9g | fiber: 2.0g | sodium: 3mg

Berry and Rhubarb Cobbler

Prep time: 15 minutes | Cook time: 35 minutes | Serves 8

Cobbler:

1 cup fresh raspberries

2 cups fresh blueberries

1 cup sliced (½-inch) rhubarb pieces

1 tablespoon arrowroot powder

¼ cup unsweetened apple juice

2 tablespoons melted coconut oil

¼ cup raw honey

Topping:

1 cup almond flour

1 tablespoon arrowroot powder

½ cup shredded coconut

¼ cup raw honey

½ cup coconut oil

Make the Cobbler

1. Preheat the oven to 350ºF (180ºC). Grease a baking dish with melted coconut oil.
2. Combine the ingredients for the cobbler in a large bowl. Stir to mix well.

3. Spread the mixture in the single layer on the baking dish. Set aside.

Make the Topping

4. Combine the almond flour, arrowroot powder, and coconut in a bowl. Stir to mix well.
5. Fold in the honey and coconut oil. Stir with a fork until the mixture crumbled.
6. Spread the topping over the cobbler, then bake in the preheated oven for 35 minutes or until frothy and golden brown.
7. Serve immediately.

Per Serving

calories: 305 | fat: 22.1g | protein: 3.2g | carbs: 29.8g | fiber: 4.0g | sodium: 3mg

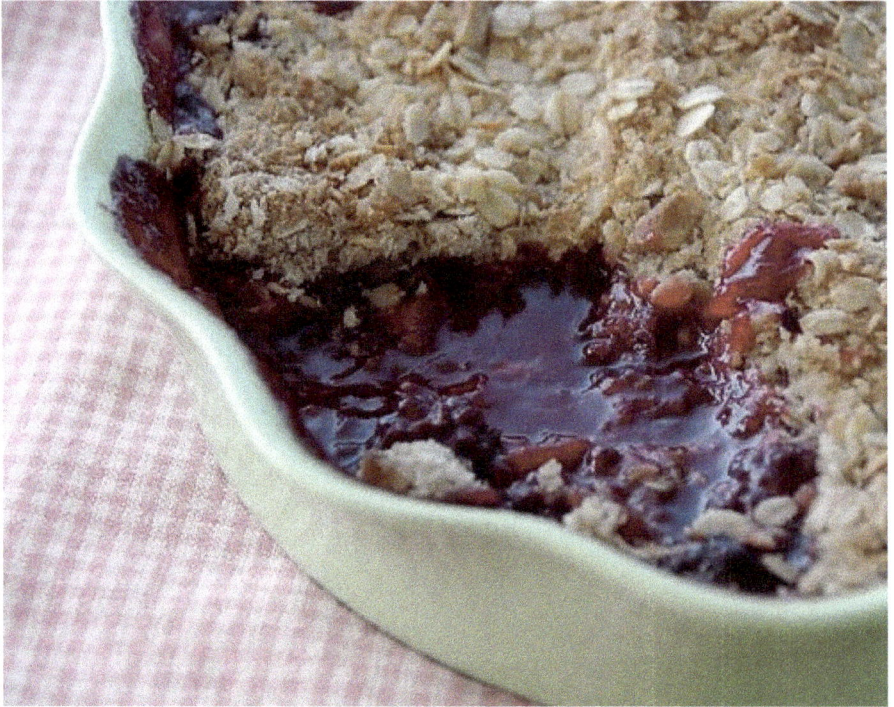

Citrus Cranberry and Quinoa Energy Bites

Prep time: 25 minutes | Cook time: 0 minutes | Makes 12 bites

2 tablespoons almond butter

2 tablespoons maple syrup

¾ cup cooked quinoa

1 tablespoon dried cranberries

1 tablespoon chia seeds

¼ cup ground almonds

¼ cup sesame seeds, toasted

Zest of 1 orange

½ teaspoon vanilla extract

1. Line a baking sheet with parchment paper.
2. Combine the butter and maple syrup in a bowl. Stir to mix well.
3. Fold in the remaining ingredients and stir until the mixture holds together and smooth.
4. Divide the mixture into 12 equal parts, then shape each part into a ball.
5. Arrange the balls on the baking sheet, then refrigerate for at least 15 minutes.

6. Serve chilled.

Per Serving (1 bite)

calories: 110 | fat: 10.8g | protein: 3.1g | carbs: 4.9g |
fiber: 3.0g | sodium: 211mg

www.ingramcontent.com/pod-product-compliance
Lightning Source LLC
Chambersburg PA
CBHW070735030426
42336CB00013B/1978